I0774795

Beginner's Guide to Anti-Inflammatory Cookbooks In 2024

Disclaimer

This book's content is solely intended for general, informative purposes. It's not the same as expert guidance. Any repercussions arising from the use or misuse of the material included herein are not the responsibility of the author or publisher. For situation-specific guidance, readers should speak with the relevant professionals. The information in the book is based on the author's knowledge as of the publishing date; any new information may not have been taken into consideration. No responsibility is assumed by the author or publisher for any mistakes, inaccuracies, or omissions. Whenever you apply concepts or advice from this book, always exercise caution and consult with knowledgeable professionals.

TABLE OF CONTENT

INTRODUCTION

<u>The Meaning of an Anti-Inflammatory Diet and Its Significance</u>

With so many inflammatory disorders and chronic illnesses around the globe, the idea of an anti-inflammatory diet has drawn a lot of interest due to its potential to improve overall health and wellbeing. The main idea behind this dietary strategy is to eat foods that have been demonstrated to lower inflammation levels in the body. In this investigation, we explore the meaning, tenets, and significant significance of implementing an anti-inflammatory diet.

What an Anti-Inflammatory Diet Is:

Choosing foods that can reduce inflammation, which is the body's natural reaction to injury, is the foundation of an anti-inflammatory diet. Since inflammation is the body's defense against damage, illness, and poisons, it is not intrinsically dangerous. On the other hand, chronic inflammation, which is defined by an ongoing immune response, is associated with a number of illnesses, such as diabetes, autoimmune diseases, cancer, and heart problems.

By restoring equilibrium to the body, an anti-inflammatory diet aims to lower chronic inflammation and improve general health. It entails consuming a diet high in anti-inflammatory foods while reducing or avoiding items that aggravate inflammation. The focus is on a sustainable, all-encompassing approach to eating that takes into account long- and short-term health benefits.

Important Anti-Inflammatory Dietary Guidelines:

1. Emphasis on Whole Foods: Eating a diet low in inflammation means consuming more whole, unprocessed foods. This diet's cornerstones include fruits, vegetables, whole grains, lean proteins, and healthy fats.

2. Omega-3 Fatty Acids: An anti-inflammatory diet should include foods high in omega-3 fatty acids, such as walnuts, flaxseeds, chia seeds, and fatty fish (salmon, mackerel, and sardines). It has been demonstrated that these lipids have strong anti-inflammatory properties.

3. Colorful Plant-Based Foods: Phytonutrients, antioxidants, and anti-inflammatory substances are indicated by the vivid colors of fruits and vegetables. A wide variety of vibrant plant-based foods offer a range of health advantages.

4. Spices and herbs:

In addition to being flavor enhancers, herbs and spices also have strong anti-inflammatory properties. There is evidence that certain foods, including cinnamon, ginger, garlic, and turmeric, have anti-inflammatory qualities.

5. Trim Proteins:

Selecting lean protein sources promotes muscular health without having the pro-inflammatory effects of some high-fat meats. Examples of these sources are fish, chicken, lentils, and plant-based proteins.

6. Reducing the amount of processed food:

An anti-inflammatory diet limits processed foods, which are frequently heavy in harmful fats, additives, and refined sugars. These products are swapped out for ones that are high in nutrients because they are known to cause inflammation.

7.Proper Macronutrient Balance:

It is crucial to maintain a balance between fats, proteins, and carbs. The emphasis is on consuming whole grains rather than refined carbohydrates and adding healthy fats like those in avocados and olive oil.

The Value of a Diet Low in Inflammations

1. Reduction of Chronic Inflammation: A number of chronic diseases share chronic inflammation as a common factor. By addressing this underlying reason, an anti-inflammatory diet may lower the chance of developing diseases like diabetes, heart disease, arthritis, and some types of cancer.

2. Cardiovascular Health: Research has linked improved cardiovascular health to the adoption of an anti-inflammatory diet. This diet lowers the risk of heart disease by decreasing inflammatory indicators and encouraging healthy blood vessel function.

3. Management of Autoimmune Illnesses: An anti-inflammatory diet may help control symptoms in those with autoimmune illnesses where the body attacks its own tissues. It may be able to mitigate some of the

hyperactivity of the immune system by lowering general inflammation.

4. Controlling Weight:

Obesity and chronic inflammation are related, and vice versa. By encouraging the consumption of nutrient-dense foods, enhancing satiety, and lowering inflammation linked to excess body fat, an anti-inflammatory diet helps manage weight.

5. Combined Health:

An anti-inflammatory diet can help with inflammatory arthritis disorders, including rheumatoid arthritis. Antioxidants and foods high in omega-3 fatty acids may help control symptoms and enhance joint health.

6. Gut Health in Balance:

Immune system performance is significantly influenced by the gut, and a healthy gut flora is supported by an anti-inflammatory diet. This in turn has a good impact on general health and may lower the likelihood of gastrointestinal problems.

7. Mental Process:

There may be a link between chronic inflammation and cognitive deterioration, according to recent studies. A diet high in antioxidants and omega-3 fatty acids that reduces inflammation may help preserve cognitive function and lower the incidence of neurodegenerative illnesses.

8. Improved Emotion and Mental Well-Being:

The link between the stomach and the brain is becoming increasingly evident, and eating an anti-inflammatory diet may have a good effect on mental health. Some meals, such as dark leafy greens and fatty fish, are linked to a lower chance of sadness and an enhanced mood.

9. Support for antioxidants:

An anti-inflammatory diet includes a lot of foods high in antioxidants. By counteracting free radicals in the body, these substances lessen oxidative stress and promote the general health of the cells.

10. Prevention of Lifestyle-Related Diseases: Adopting an anti-inflammatory diet can help reduce the risk of lifestyle-related diseases, which are frequently linked to poor dietary choices. By addressing the underlying

causes of inflammation, people can either manage or avoid these illnesses.

In summary:

In summary, an anti-inflammatory diet is a scientifically supported strategy with significant benefits for health and wellbeing, not just a gastronomic fad. People who comprehend and adopt the tenets of this dietary approach may be able to lessen the effects of chronic inflammation and lower their chance of developing a number of illnesses.

How Nutritional Decisions Affect Inflammation

Dietary decisions become a potent thread in the complex web of our health, one that can either contribute to the complex pattern of inflammation or tell a story of well-being. When inflammation changes from a temporary reaction to a chronic condition, it might pose a threat to health. Inflammation is a normal and necessary defensive mechanism. More and more research is pointing to chronic inflammation as a risk factor for a wide range of illnesses, including autoimmune diseases, neurological disorders, and metabolic and cardiovascular diseases.

Knowing how food interacts with inflammation reveals a world in which food is information that interacts with our cells and affects the complex dance of the immune system, rather than only providing nourishment. This investigation explores the processes through which dietary decisions affect inflammation, the function of particular nutrients, and the significant consequences for general health.

The Changing Relationship Between Food Selection and Inflammation

Fundamentally, inflammation is the body's reaction to damage, infection, or negative stimuli. This protective mechanism, known as acute inflammation, works to remove injured cells, stop the source of cell injury, and start the healing process of damaged tissue. But if this process continues too long or gets out of control, it develops chronic inflammation and can lead to a host of other health problems.

The fine balance between the body's pro- and anti-inflammatory signals is mostly controlled by dietary decisions. The kinds of food we eat affect the synthesis of chemicals that are either pro- or anti-inflammatory, which affects our immune system and the inflammatory environment as a whole. This dynamic link can be attributed to several important factors:

1. The composition of nutrients:

Our diet's macronutrient makeup, particularly the ratio of proteins, fats, and carbs, has a significant impact on inflammation. Diets heavy in unhealthy fats and processed carbohydrates have been connected to higher levels of inflammatory markers; on the other hand, diets high in fiber, antioxidants, and omega-3 fatty acids have been linked to anti-inflammatory benefits.

2. The gut microbiota

The trillions of bacteria called the gut microbiota that live in our digestive tracts are essential for controlling inflammation. Dietary decisions support a varied and well-balanced microbiota, especially those high in fiber and plant-based meals. The generation of anti-inflammatory chemicals and immune system modulation are facilitated by a healthy gut microbiome.

3. Phytonutrients and antioxidants:

Antioxidants and phytonutrients are abundant in fruits, vegetables, herbs, and spices. Free radicals are reactive chemicals that cause inflammation and oxidative stress. These substances counteract them. Eating a wide variety of colored plant-based foods offers strong resistance against inflammatory processes.

4. The Fatty Acids Omega-3:

Omega-3 fatty acids are well known for their anti-inflammatory qualities. They are mostly present in walnuts, flaxseeds, chia seeds, and fatty fish. By acting as building blocks for anti-inflammatory compounds, these vital fats assist in regulating the inflammatory response.

5. Foods and additives processed:

Foods that have been processed and are frequently high in harmful fats, refined sugars, and additives are linked to systemic inflammation. These food ingredients have the potential to cause inflammation and upset the immune system's delicate balance.

6. Foods Fermented and Probiotics:

Fermented foods such as yogurt, kefir, and sauerkraut include probiotics, which are good microorganisms that promote intestinal health. These foods support a gut flora that is in a healthy state, which reduces inflammation.

7. Immunological-modulating minerals: A number of minerals, including zinc, vitamin D, and vitamin E, are crucial for immunological function. Insufficiency in these nutrients may weaken the immune system and perhaps increase inflammation.

Comprehending how dietary decisions affect inflammation requires a sophisticated understanding of the complex biochemical reactions that occur in our bodies as a result of the foods we eat. Let's now explore in more detail the particular foods and dietary habits that either exacerbate or reduce inflammation.

Particular Nutrients and How They Affect Inflammation

1. Omega-3 Fatty Acids: Eicosapentaenoic acid (EPA) and docosahexaenoic acid (DHA) are two examples of omega-3 fatty acids that have strong anti-inflammatory properties. These fats, which may be found in plant-based foods like flaxseeds and walnuts as well as fatty

fish like salmon and mackerel, act as building blocks for molecules that reduce inflammation.

2. Antioxidants: Antioxidants, such as beta-carotene, selenium, and the vitamins C and E, neutralize free radicals and lessen oxidative stress. Antioxidants are abundant in fruits (strawberries, citrus fruits), vegetables (carrots, leafy greens), and nuts (sunflower seeds, almonds).

3. Polyphenols:

Rich in dark chocolate, tea, coffee, and many fruits and vegetables, polyphenols have antioxidant and anti-inflammatory qualities. These substances improve general health by regulating inflammatory pathways.

4. Fiber:

Dietary fiber has anti-inflammatory properties and is found in whole grains, legumes, fruits, and vegetables. Fiber helps to regulate immunological responses, fosters the growth of good bacteria in the gut, and improves gut health.

5. Probiotics:

Probiotics improve the diversity of the gut microbiota and are present in fermented foods such as kimchi, sauerkraut, kefir, and yogurt. Improved immunological response and decreased inflammation are linked to a balanced gut flora.

6. Curcumin and Turmeric:

Spices like turmeric, which contain the active ingredient curcumin, are well known for their strong anti-inflammatory and antioxidant qualities. Since curcumin modifies inflammatory pathways, it is a useful supplement to a diet that reduces inflammation.

7. Vitamin D

Vitamin D is involved in immunological regulation and can be derived from sunshine, fatty fish, and fortified meals. Reduced inflammation and a decreased chance of developing autoimmune diseases are linked to adequate vitamin D levels.

8. Zinc

Lean meats, nuts, seeds, and legumes are good sources of zinc, which also has anti-inflammatory properties and boosts immunity.

The mechanisms by which diet affects inflammation are:

Investigating the molecular interactions inside our body's complex systems is necessary to comprehend the ways in which dietary choices impact inflammation. In these processes, a number of important routes and mediators are important players.

1. The NF-κB Pathway One important transcription factor implicated in inflammation is nuclear factor-kappa B (NF-κB). Foods that promote inflammation, like those heavy in sugar and saturated fats, can trigger the activation of NF-κB, which in turn causes the release of inflammatory mediators and cytokines.

2. Oxidative Stress: An imbalance between the body's capacity to neutralize free radicals and their creation is the result of unhealthy dietary patterns. Inflammation is brought on by oxidative stress, which is also linked to a number of chronic illnesses.

3. Influence of the Gut Microbiota: Immune modulation is greatly influenced by the gut microbiota, a diverse

colony of bacteria in the digestive system. Dietary decisions, especially those high in fiber and prebiotics, affect inflammation by modifying the makeup and functionality of the gut microbiota.

4. Pro-Resolving Mediators: A few food ingredients, particularly omega-3 fatty acids, help the body produce pro-resolving mediators. These specific molecules actively work to resolve inflammation and stop it from lasting over time.

5. Foods high in antioxidants and anti-inflammatory substances can promote the generation of cytokines that have anti-inflammatory characteristics. These cytokines aid in the control of immunological responses and the reduction of inflammation.

advantages of having a non-inflammatory lifestyle

There are numerous advantages to living an anti-inflammatory lifestyle that affect one's physical, mental, and general health. Here's a quick rundown of the main benefits:

1. Decreased Chronic Inflammation: People can lessen chronic inflammation, a frequent underlying cause of

many chronic diseases, by adopting anti-inflammatory dietary choices. Thus, there is a decreased chance of developing ailments, including diabetes, heart disease, and some autoimmune diseases.

2. Enhancement of Cardiovascular Health: By lowering inflammation and enhancing parameters like cholesterol and blood vessel function, an anti-inflammatory lifestyle promotes cardiovascular health. This encourages a healthier circulatory system and reduces the risk of heart illness.

3. Assistance with Weight Management:

Adopting anti-inflammatory behaviors, such as a balanced diet and frequent exercise, helps manage weight since chronic inflammation is associated with obesity. For general health, it's important to maintain a healthy weight.

4. Enhancing Joint Health:

An anti-inflammatory lifestyle can help people with inflammatory joint disorders such as arthritis manage their symptoms and maintain the health of their joints.

Antioxidants and foods high in omega-3 fatty acids may help to lessen joint inflammation.

5. Enhanced Digestive Health

Immune modulation is significantly influenced by the gut microbiota, and a lifestyle low in inflammation promotes a diversified and well-balanced gut microbiome. This encourages the best possible gut health, nutrient absorption, and digestion.

6. A balanced level of blood sugar:

Stable blood sugar levels are a result of anti-inflammatory dietary choices, such as emphasizing natural foods over processed and sugary options. This is especially helpful for people who are managing or at risk of diabetes.

7. Improved mental well-being:

There may be a connection between mental health issues and inflammation, according to recent studies. With its focus on nutrient-rich foods and antioxidants, an anti-inflammatory diet may enhance mood and lower the chance of developing diseases like depression.

8. Reduced Chance of Chronic Illnesses:

Many diseases have chronic inflammatory disorders as a prelude. People can proactively lower their chance of developing chronic diseases and maintain long-term health by leading an anti-inflammatory lifestyle.

9. Enhanced Vitality:

Long-lasting energy is provided by nutrient-dense meals that are a component of an anti-inflammatory diet. This is in contrast to the swings in energy that are frequently linked to diets high in harmful fats and processed carbohydrates.

10. bolstering the immune system

An anti-inflammatory, well-balanced lifestyle helps the immune system function better and fight off infections and other problems. This holds special significance for resilience and general well-being.

11. Improved Quality of Sleep:

Sleep difficulties have been connected to chronic inflammation. Reducing inflammation in the body by practicing relaxation techniques and eating foods that promote sleep can help with both general sleep patterns and the quality of sleep.

12. Lifespan and Well-Being Aging:

A lifestyle low in inflammation promotes good aging by lessening the negative effects of chronic inflammation on the body. Preventing age-related illnesses and promoting overall longevity.

13. Support for Cancer Prevention: Although adopting an anti-inflammatory lifestyle, which includes a diet high in antioxidants and anti-inflammatory chemicals, does not ensure that cancer will not develop, it may lessen the risk of developing some types of cancer.

14. Enhanced Cognitive Function: Neurodegenerative disorders and cognitive loss are linked to chronic inflammation. A diet high in antioxidants and omega-3 fatty acids, as well as an anti-inflammatory lifestyle, may improve cognitive performance and lower the risk of diseases like Alzheimer's.

15. Beneficial Effect on Skin Health: A number of skin disorders are influenced by inflammation. Living an anti-

inflammatory lifestyle could help you have a healthier complexion, less redness, and smoother skin.

Adopting an anti-inflammatory lifestyle is, in essence, a comprehensive approach to health that goes beyond simple dietary modifications. It emphasizes the complex relationships between diet, exercise, mental health, and illness prevention, encompassing total well-being. Such a lifestyle can be an empowered and proactive step toward long-term health goals.

UNDERSTANDING INFLAMMATION

A Comprehensive Examination of Acute and Chronic Inflammation

The body uses inflammation, a complicated and dynamic biological reaction, to protect itself against dangerous stimuli, including infections, wounds, and irritants. This process is highly regulated and comprises a complex cascade of molecular and cellular events with the goals of removing the harmful source, removing damaged cells, and starting the healing process of the tissue. It's critical to distinguish between acute and chronic inflammation in order to comprehend the two basic forms of inflammation.Acute Inflammation

Acute inflammation is the body's first, fast reaction to an injury or infection. It is a quick, focused procedure that seeks to both start the healing process and neutralize and eradicate the causing agent. The body needs acute inflammation as a defense mechanism in order to survive and heal.

Important attributes:

1. Fast Onset: Acute inflammation starts as soon as the harmful stimulus is initiated. The objective of the quick response is to neutralize the threat as soon as possible.

2. Minimal Length: Acute inflammation usually has a minimal length, ranging from several hours to several

days. The process ends when the threat is eliminated and the damaged tissues recover to their original state.

3. Vasodilation and Increased Permeability: As a result of the affected area's blood vessel dilatation, blood flow is enhanced. The blood artery walls become more permeable as a result, making it possible for immune cells and proteins to get to the site of an injury or infection.

4. Cellular Infiltration: To get rid of the threat, white blood cells—mainly neutrophils—move to the damaged area. These cells take up and eliminate infections or clear debris from damaged tissues.

5. Classic Indication Indicators: Heat, Redness, Swelling, and Pain: During acute inflammation, these classic indicators of inflammation are visible. Increased blood flow, immune cell activity, and healing processes are all indicated by these symptoms.

6. Resolution and Tissue Repair: Anti-inflammatory signals initiate the resolution phase when the threat has been eliminated. This entails tissue repair, immune cell elimination, and the return of normal function.

The body uses acute inflammation as a helpful and strictly controlled defense mechanism against impending danger. It is critical for preserving tissue homeostasis and is part of the immune response.

Prolonged Inflammation:

The term "chronic inflammation" refers to an inflammatory reaction that lasts for a long time, perhaps from weeks to years. Chronic inflammation can be harmful to tissues and is linked to a number of chronic diseases, in contrast to acute inflammation, which is a protective and self-limiting process.

Important attributes:

  1. Long-TDuration: Chronic inflammation lasts for a long time, and the resolution stage might not be finished. This prolonged reaction may result in ongoing tissue damage and malfunction.

2. Immune Cell Infiltration: Compared to acute inflammation, the makeup of immune cells in chronic inflammation is different. In chronic inflammatory situations, monocytes, macrophages, and lymphocytes are more common.

3. Attempts at Tissue Destruction and Repair

Both attempts at healing and tissue damage can result from persistent inflammation. Prolonged immune cell and inflammatory mediator presence contributes to tissue architectural disruption and persistent damage.

4. Development of Granulomas:

Granulomas, which are arranged clusters of immune cells, can develop in some chronic inflammatory diseases, such as sarcoidosis or tuberculosis, as the body tries to contain recurring threats.

5. Systemic Repercussions:

Chronic inflammation frequently has systemic effects, in contrast to acute inflammation. Released into the bloodstream, inflammatory mediators can impact distant organs and tissues, which can aid in the development of systemic diseases.

6. Connections to Long-Term Illnesses:

Numerous chronic diseases, including diabetes, autoimmune disorders, neurodegenerative diseases, cardiovascular diseases, and several types of cancer, are linked to chronic inflammation. It may affect general health and hasten the course of various disorders.

Chronic inflammation's causes include:

Prolonged exposure to irritants (like tobacco smoke), autoimmune illnesses (where the immune system mistakenly targets the body's own tissues), situations like obesity (where extra adipose tissue generates pro-inflammatory signals), and persistent infections can all lead to chronic inflammation.

Identifying Characteristics:

The classic four of symptoms associated with acute inflammation—heat, redness, swelling, and pain—are absent from chronic inflammation. As opposed to this, it frequently manifests as a low-grade, simmering process with **less obvious symptoms.**

Knowing the distinctions between acute and chronic inflammation is essential for our understanding of disease processes as well as clinical settings. While chronic inflammation, when left unchecked, can contribute to the onset and progression of a wide range of crippling diseases, acute inflammation is a protective and adaptive response.

An Extensive Examination of the Function of Inflammation in Different Medical Disorders

An essential component of the immune system, inflammation has two functions for human health. Acute inflammation is a protective, localized reaction that is essential for healing and protection against pathogens, while persistent inflammation is linked to the etiology and development of many diseases. This talk examines the complex role that inflammation plays in a number of medical problems, including autoimmune diseases, neurological disorders, metabolic diseases, and cardiovascular diseases.

- Heart-related Conditions:
  ★ Atherosclerosis:

Inflammatory Trigger: The development of atherosclerosis, a disorder marked by the accumulation of plaque in arteries, is largely caused by chronic inflammation.

Mechanism: Fatty deposits in vascular walls are facilitated by inflammatory mediators, which also draw immune cells that worsen the development of plaque. Heart attacks and strokes can result from blood clots formed as a result of inflammation-induced plaque rupture.

★ Heart Failure:

Inflammatory Response: Heart failure is linked to persistent inflammation. Fibrosis, decreased contractility, and cardiac remodeling are all influenced by inflammatory signals.Cytokine Involvement: Heart failure patients have higher than normal concentrations of pro-inflammatory cytokines such as TNF-alpha and IL-6.

- Disorders of Metabolism:

★Diabetes Type 2:

Insulin Resistance: Insulin resistance is a hallmark of type 2 diabetes and is associated with chronic inflammation, particularly in adipose tissue.Impact of Cytokines: Pro-inflammatory cytokines secreted by adipose tissue impede insulin signaling and stimulate systemic inflammation.

★Overweight:

Adipose Tissue Inflammation: Chronic inflammation of the adipose tissue in obese people results in the release of inflammatory chemicals.   Insulin Resistance and Comorbidities: Insulin resistance is influenced by inflammatory signals, and comorbidities such as cardiovascular illnesses are associated with inflammation related to obesity.

Conditions Caused by Autoimmune Response:

- Diabetic arthritis:
★Synovial Inflammation: Rheumatoid arthritis patients experience joint discomfort, swelling, and damage as a result of synovial inflammation.Immune System Dysfunction: The immune system attacks joint tissues as a result of autoimmune reactions, which prolong inflammation.
★IBDs, or inflammatory bowel diseases:

Chronic inflammation of the gastrointestinal tract is a feature of diseases such as Crohn's disease and ulcerative colitis.Immunological dysregulation: When immunological responses are out of control, the intestinal lining is harmed, which causes symptoms including diarrhea and stomach pain.

- Neurodegenerative Conditions:

★Alzheimer's illness:

Neuroinflammation: Alzheimer's disease is linked to persistent inflammation in the brain.   Activation of Microglia: Inflammatory chemicals are released by activated microglia, which leads to neuronal injury and cognitive impairment.

★Parkinson's illness:

Inflammatory Component: Parkinson's disease development is linked to inflammation.   Activation of Microglia: Neurodegeneration is facilitated by the production of pro-inflammatory chemicals by activated microglia.

- Cancer:

The Risk of Cancer with Chronic Inflammation:

★Inflammatory Microenvironment: Prolonged inflammation has been connected to the onset and spread of several malignancies.

★Promotion of Tumor Development: An environment that is favorable to tumor development and metastasis can be produced by inflammatory signals.

- Long-Term Respiratory Disorders:

COPD stands for chronic obstructive pulmonary disease.

★Airway Inflammation: One of the main characteristics of COPD is a persistent inflammation of the airways.   Effect on Lung Function: Airflow restriction and anatomical alterations in the lungs are caused by inflammatory reactions.

★Having asthma:

Airway Inflammation: The symptoms of asthma are partly caused by a persistent inflammation of the airways.Immune cells have a key role in bronchoconstriction and hyperresponsive airways by releasing inflammatory mediators.

- Renal Inflammation in Chronic Kidney Disease Persistent inflammation is a feature of chronic renal disease as kidney damage progresses. Inflammatory Mediators: Cytokines and other inflammatory compounds are linked to renal impairment and fibrosis.

- The Aging Process in Part:Aging and Inflammation:igniting Chronic, low-grade inflammation contributes to age-related diseases and is associated with aging. Cellular Senescence: The inflammatory response is linked to the process of cellular senescence, which affects tissue repair and function.

- Autoimmune syndromes:Genetic Conditions: Autoinflammatory disorders are the result of dysregulated inflammatory responses brought on by genetic abnormalities. Unprovoked Inflammation: Unprovoked inflammation episodes are common in people with autoinflammatory illnesses.

Skin Conditions That Cause Inflammation:

1. psoriasis:

Immune-Mediated Inflammation: An inflammatory response on the skin is a hallmark of psoriasis. Cytokines: The chronic nature of the illness and skin lesions are caused by increased amounts of pro-inflammatory cytokines.

2. Atopic dermatitis, or eczema:

Immune Response in the Skin: Eczema is characterized by a persistent inflammatory response to stimuli.   Skin Barrier Dysfunction: Flare-ups can result from inflammatory processes that compromise the skin barrier.

Influence on Mental Well-Being:

3. Depression

Inflammatory Markers: People with depression are more likely to have elevated levels of inflammatory markers due to chronic inflammation. Neuroinflammation: Neurochemical abnormalities associated with depressed symptoms may be exacerbated by inflammation in the brain.

4. Disorders of Anxiety:

Inflammatory Factors: Anxiety-related neurotransmitter systems may be impacted by inflammatory processes.   Interaction with the Nervous System: Activation of the immune system may have an impact on the central nervous system, which may lead to symptoms associated with anxiety.

In summary:

Although inflammation plays a crucial role in the immune response, it is persistent and dysregulated inflammation that lies at the root of many diseases. Comprehending the complex interactions among the immune system, inflammatory reactions, and particular ailments is essential for formulating focused treatment strategies and measures. Immunology is a dynamic subject that is constantly deciphering the intricate nature of inflammation and providing fresh perspectives on possible approaches to treating a variety of medical ailments.

<u>The Significance of Managing Inflammation via Nutritional Decisions</u>

An essential component of the body's defense system, inflammation has two drawbacks. Acute inflammation is an essential reaction to wounds and infections, but persistent inflammation is associated with a wide range of medical conditions. Understanding how food choices affect inflammation has grown in importance since it provides a proactive and approachable means of enhancing general health and averting chronic illnesses. The following main points emphasize how crucial it is to manage inflammation through dietary decisions:

1. Prevention of Chronic Diseases:

Many chronic diseases, such as diabetes, heart disease, and some types of cancer, have chronic inflammation as a common denominator. By implementing an anti-inflammatory diet high in fruits, vegetables, and omega-3 fatty acids, one may be able to lessen the chance of developing chronic inflammation and related illnesses.

2. Heart Health:

An important factor in the start and development of atherosclerosis, a disorder marked by the accumulation of plaque in arteries, is inflammation. By reducing the likelihood of plaque development and enhancing overall vascular function, dietary choices that minimize inflammation, such as including antioxidants and healthy fats, improve cardiovascular health.3. 3. Health of the Metabolic Process:

Obesity and other metabolic diseases, like insulin resistance, are closely linked to inflammation. Selecting blood sugar-stabilizing meals, like lean proteins and whole grains, can aid in the management and prevention of many disorders by improving metabolic health and lowering inflammatory markers.

4. Mutual Health:

An anti-inflammatory diet can help those with inflammatory joint diseases such as rheumatoid arthritis. Certain meals, like those high in antioxidants and omega-3 fatty acids, may enhance general joint health by reducing joint pain and swelling.

5. Digestive Health:

Immune modulation is greatly influenced by the gut microbiota, and disruptions in gut health may be a factor in long-term inflammation. A varied and healthy gut flora is fostered by a diet rich in fiber and probiotics, which improve digestive health and reduce inflammation.

6. Control of Weight:

Obesity and persistent low-grade inflammation are frequently linked. Reducing inflammation and enhancing general health can be achieved by adopting dietary choices that assist weight control, such as placing an emphasis on whole, nutrient-dense meals and minimizing processed and sugary goods.

7. Physiological Health:

Numerous neurological illnesses, such as Parkinson's and Alzheimer's, are linked to inflammation. Foods high in antioxidants and those with anti-inflammatory qualities, including fatty fish and turmeric, may promote cognitive function and have neuroprotective effects.

8. Immune System Assistance:

Foods high in nutrients support a healthy immune system. Sufficient consumption of vitamins, minerals, and antioxidants boosts the immune system, enabling the body to fight infections and lower the risk of long-term inflammation.

9. Skin Conditions:

Skin diseases like psoriasis, acne, and eczema can be impacted by inflammatory processes. Clearer skin and a healthier complexion may be the result of some dietary choices, particularly those that have anti-inflammatory qualities.

10. Mental Wellness:

Recent studies point to a connection between mental health issues, including anxiety, depression, and inflammation. A nutrient-rich diet may help to promote emotional well-being, even if it cannot completely replace comprehensive mental health measures.

11. Extended-Term Welfare:

Reducing inflammation with nutrition is an investment in long-term health, not just a way to handle present health problems. People who lead anti-inflammatory lifestyles may age more gracefully, experience fewer age-related illnesses, and have a higher quality of life overall.

In summary:

It is crucial to reduce inflammation through food, and this cannot be emphasized enough. An intelligent and deliberate approach to eating can significantly affect the inflammatory state of the body, affecting the body's resistance to disease and fostering vitality. Although dietary decisions are not a cure-all, they are a strong and useful tool that people may use to actively participate in their health and wellbeing. As they say, "Let food be thy medicine," highlighting the significant impact that our dietary decisions can have on the complex interplay between inflammation and health.

BASICS OF AN ANTI-INFLAMMATORY DIET

Essential Elements and Guidelines for an Anti-Inflammatory Diet

An anti-inflammatory diet is based on eating choices that try to lessen the body's chronic inflammation, which is a major contributing factor to the onset of many chronic illnesses. The following is a summary of the main ideas and elements of an anti-inflammatory diet:1. A focus on whole foods derived from plants:

1. Fruits and vegetables: The cornerstone of any anti-inflammatory diet is a diet rich in antioxidants, vitamins, and minerals. They support the fight against oxidative stress and free radicals.Leafy Greens: Leafy greens like spinach, kale, and others are very high in chemicals that reduce inflammation, so incorporate them on a daily basis.

2. Omega-3 Fatty Acids and Good Fats:

Fatty Fish: Rich in omega-3 fatty acids, which are believed to have anti-inflammatory qualities, salmon, mackerel, and sardines are good sources of fat. The ratio of omega-6 to omega-3 in the diet is aided by these fats.Nuts and Seeds: Rich in omega-3 fatty acids and other nutrients that promote a healthy inflammatory response, walnuts, flaxseeds, and chia seeds.

3. Complete Grains:

Quinoa, Brown Rice, and Oats: Whole grains give you minerals and fiber that support gut health and help control blood sugar, which lowers inflammatory risk.

4. Vegetables:

Chickpeas, lentils, and beans are examples of legumes that are high in plant-based protein and fiber. They encourage a varied gut flora and have anti-inflammatory properties.

5. Trim Proteins:

Fish, poultry, and plant-based proteins: Selecting lean protein sources can help lower consumption of saturated fat. Legumes, fish, and plant-based proteins like tofu are particularly healthy.

6. Spices and herbs:

Curcumin, a strong anti-inflammatory substance, is found in turmeric. It may be helpful for a number of medical disorders and has been linked to decreased inflammation.Ginger: This versatile ingredient can be used in both savory and sweet recipes because of its anti-inflammatory and antioxidant qualities.

7. Nutritious Cooking Fats:

Extra virgin olive oil, which contains monounsaturated fats with anti-inflammatory properties, is a mainstay of the Mediterranean diet.Avocado Oil: Packed with antioxidants and monounsaturated fats, avocado oil can be cooked at higher temperatures.

Probiotics and Foods with Fermentation:

Probiotics found in yogurt, kefir, and kimchi help maintain intestinal health. Decreased inflammation is associated with a varied and well-balanced gut microbiome.

9. Anti-inflammatory and colorful foods:

Berries: Packed with antioxidants and polyphenols, blueberries, strawberries, and raspberries have anti-inflammatory properties.Dark Chocolate: Flavonoids found in dark chocolate with a high cocoa content may have anti-inflammatory properties when consumed in moderation.

10. Cutting Back on Processed Foods:

Steer clear of added sugars. Sugar-filled drinks and processed foods can aggravate inflammation. One of the main components of an anti-inflammatory diet is reducing added sugar intake.Limiting Refined Carbohydrates: Consuming white bread and other refined carbs can cause blood sugar to increase, which may worsen inflammation.

11. Drink plenty of water.

Water and herbal teas: Maintaining proper hydration is critical to general health. Hydration is aided by herbal teas and water that don't have any added caffeine or sugar.

12. Balance and Moderation:

Portion Control: Eating in moderation lowers the risk of inflammation linked to obesity and helps with weight management by preventing overeating.A varied diet guarantees a wide spectrum of nutrients, promoting general health and a well-regulated inflammatory response.

13. Individualization

Customized Approach: Understanding that everyone has different nutritional requirements, an anti-inflammatory diet can be tailored to an individual's age, health, and preferences, among other things.

Items on an Anti-Inflammatory Diet to Steer Clear of:

1. Processed Foods: Steer clear of packaged foods with extra sweets and harmful fats, fast meals, and processed snacks. These may be a factor in inflammation.

2. Sugar Added: Steer clear of sugar-filled drinks, sweets, and pastries. Consuming too much sugar might cause inflammation and other metabolic problems.

3. Refined Carbs: Steer clear of pastries, white bread, and other refined carbs. These may result in blood sugar surges, which will fuel inflammation.

4. Saturated and Trans Fats: Steer clear of foods heavy in trans fats, fried foods, and red and processed meats. These lipids may be involved in cardiovascular problems and inflammation.

5. Extensively Manicured Oils:

Steer clear of cooking oils with a lot of omega-6 fatty acids, like soybean and corn oil. In order to lower inflammation, omega-3 and omega-6 fatty acids must be in equilibrium.

6. Drinking too much alcohol:

Steer clear of excessive alcohol intake, as this can exacerbate inflammation and have a detrimental effect on general health.

7. Synthetic Additives:

Foods containing artificial coloring, preservatives, and additives should be avoided. In certain people, they might be a factor in inflammation and allergic reactions.

8. Overindulgence in Salt:

Foods high in sodium should be avoided since too much salt can aggravate inflammation and raise the risk of hypertension.

9. Meats that have been processed:

Sausage, bacon, and other processed meats should be avoided. These are loaded with harmful fats and substances that cause inflammation.

10. Limit or Avoid dairy: People who are lactose intolerant or sensitive to dairy proteins may find that cutting back on their dairy consumption helps reduce inflammation.

11. Nightshade Vegetables: Limit: Because nightshade vegetables like tomatoes, peppers, and eggplants might aggravate symptoms, some people with specific inflammatory disorders may decide to limit their intake of these foods.

12. Gluten: Limit or Avoid: Steer clear of gluten-containing grains, including wheat, barley, and rye, if you have celiac disease or are sensitive to gluten. This may help minimize inflammation.

Making deliberate decisions to emphasize whole, nutrient-dense meals while reducing or avoiding processed and possibly inflammatory foods is the foundation of an anti-inflammatory diet. While adhering to these broad recommendations, it is imperative to take individual tolerance and preferences into account. Speaking with a dietician or medical expert might provide tailored guidance based on particular health needs and conditions.

In summary, an anti-inflammatory diet consists mostly of a wide variety of full, high-nutrient foods that work together to help the body's chronic inflammation. Individuals can actively contribute to their general health and well-being, possibly preventing or treating chronic inflammatory disorders, by implementing these concepts and components into their regular eating habits.

INTRODUCTION TO ANTI-INFLAMMATORY COOKING

Crucial Cooking Equipment for an Anti-Inflammatory Diet:

- Good Chef's Knife: It's easier and more efficient to cut fruits, vegetables, and other ingredients with a well-made, sharp chef's knife.
- Cutting Board: A solid cutting board offers a roomy and secure surface for chopping and dicing a wide range of foods.
- Vegetable Peeler: An excellent tool for increasing the amount of plant-based foods in your diet, a

vegetable peeler is useful for peeling fruits and vegetables.

- Grater: Adding taste and anti-inflammatory ingredients to food is possible by using a grater to grate fresh ginger, turmeric, or citrus zest.

- Garlic Press: Adding fresh garlic to your food is made easier with a garlic press, which also improves flavor and may have health advantages.

- Food processor or blender:

Perfect for blending nutrient-dense foods like fruits, vegetables, and nuts into smoothies, soups, or homemade sauces.

- Non-stick Cooking Surface:

When using a non-stick pan, you can cook lean proteins or sauté veggies with less added fat because you won't need as much cooking oil.

- Steamer Basket:

Vegetables cooked gradually with steam in a steamer basket retain more of their nutrients.

- Baking sheets:

Baking sheets come in handy for baking anti-inflammatory goodies, making kale chips, and roasting vegetables.

- Glass jars or Mason jars:

Perfect for preserving homemade dressings, sauces, and prepared foods. It is best to use glass containers to prevent any possible chemical leaching.

- Juicer with citrus:

Citrus juice that has just been squeezed can add flavor and anti-inflammatory elements. Juicing citrus fruits with a juicer is quick and easy.

- Herb Conservator:

Using an herb keeper will help you preserve the flavor and nutritional benefits of fresh herbs like parsley and cilantro for longer.

<u>Crucial Components of a Dietary Anti-Inflammatory:</u>

★Turmeric: Packed with curcumin and a strong anti-inflammatory, turmeric can be added to soups, smoothies, and curries, among other foods.

★ Ginger: Ginger, either fresh or ground, has anti-inflammatory and digestive properties and gives food a burst of flavor.

★ Extra Virgin Olive Oil: Rich in anti-inflammatory qualities and heart-healthy, extra virgin olive oil works wonders in salad dressings and low-temperature cooking.

★ Berries: You may add antioxidant-rich blueberries, strawberries, and other berries to breakfast bowls, snacks, and desserts.

★ Leafy Greens: Rich in vitamins and minerals, leafy greens such as spinach and kale are a great source of nutrition. Add them to sautés, salads, and smoothies.

★ Saturated Fish:

Sardines, mackerel, and salmon are good sources of omega-3 fatty acids. Because of their anti-inflammatory properties, include them in your diet.

★ Seeds and nuts:

Almonds, walnuts, flaxseeds, and chia seeds are good sources of anti-inflammatory and healthful fats. Add them to snacks or sprinkle them over yogurt.

★ Quinoa:

Quinoa is a multipurpose, nutrient-dense whole grain that may be used as a side dish or as a foundation for salads and bowls.

★ Trim Proteins:

Lean proteins such as lentils, tofu, and chicken are good choices for a balanced diet that doesn't contain too much saturated fat.

★ Garlic

Garlic adds flavor and may have anti-inflammatory properties that improve the flavor of many foods.

★ Green Tea:

Green tea, which is high in antioxidants, is a nutritious beverage option that may have anti-inflammatory properties.

- ★ Dark Chocolate with 70% or More Cocoa: When consumed in moderation, dark chocolate with a high cocoa content offers antioxidants and flavonoids.
- ★ Herbs and Spices: To improve flavor and provide anti-inflammatory components, add a variety of

herbs and spices, such as cinnamon, thyme, rosemary, and basil.

★ Foods High in Probiotics: Fermented foods like sauerkraut, kefir, and yogurt all improve gut health and may even reduce inflammation.

★ Whole Grains: To get fiber and other nutrients, choose whole grains such as brown rice, oats, and whole wheat.

Beginners can simply start on an anti-inflammatory diet journey and create tasty, nourishing meals that support general health and well-being by keeping these basic kitchen tools and materials on hand.

Advice on Organizing and Preparing Anti-Inflammatory Meals:

1. Give Emphasis to Whole, Plant-Based Foods: Plan your meals with an emphasis on fruits, vegetables, whole grains, legumes, and nuts. These foods offer a wide range of anti-inflammatory nutrients and antioxidants.

2. Incorporate a Range of Colors: Diverse nutrient profiles are represented by the colors of fruits and

vegetables. To guarantee a variety of anti-inflammatory chemicals, aim for a colorful dish.

3. Plan Balanced Meals: To give sustained energy and encourage satiety, make sure each meal has a balance of lean proteins, healthy fats, and complex carbohydrates.

4. Include Fatty Fish: For their omega-3 fatty acids, which are believed to have anti-inflammatory qualities, include fatty fish, such as mackerel or salmon, at least twice a week.

5. Use Anti-Inflammatory Herbs and Spices: To enhance the taste and anti-inflammatory properties of your food, try experimenting with herbs like turmeric, ginger, and garlic, as well as spices like cumin and cinnamon.

6. Make your own homemade dressings and sauces.

Use spices, herbs, and olive oil to make your own sauces and dressings. This gives you ingredient control, so you may stay away from bad fats and extra sweets.

7. Using batch cooking to save time:

Make extra servings of anti-inflammatory mainstays such as quinoa, roasted veggies, or lean proteins so you always have them on hand for easy, well-balanced meals all week long.

8. Adopt a Fermented Diet:

Include items that have undergone fermentation, such as kefir, sauerkraut, or yogurt, in your diet. These foods may reduce inflammation and support intestinal health.

9. Methods of Mindful Cooking:

Use cooking techniques like steaming, sautéing, or roasting to retain the nutritional value of your food. Reduce the amount of deep-frying and overcooking on high heat.

10. Arrange snacks in advance:

Instead of looking for commercial foods, prepare anti-inflammatory snacks like fresh fruit, almonds, or veggie sticks with hummus.

11. Maintain Hydration:

Water is your best beverage throughout the day. Staying hydrated promotes general health and helps the body continue to operate at its best, even in terms of inflammation.

12. Examine the labels on food:

Pay attention to the ingredient lists of processed foods. Steer clear of items that cause inflammation, such as those with artificial additives, bad fats, and added sweets.

13. Play Around with Different Grains:

To increase the variety of nutrients in your diet, consider including grains other than rice, such as millet, quinoa, or farro.

14. Conscious Portion Control:

To avoid overindulging, be mindful of portion proportions. By eating with awareness, you can better detect when you are full and enjoy your food.

15. Speak with an Expert in Nutrition:

Seek individualized advice from a licensed dietitian or nutritionist if you have any particular dietary issues or medical conditions.

16. Make smoothies to reduce inflammation.

Smoothies are a delightful and nutrient-dense choice when you blend fruits like berries, leafy greens, and an omega-3 source (like chia or flaxseeds) together.

17. Plan Ahead for Eating Out: Examine menus in advance and choose meals that support your anti-inflammatory objectives. Choose salads, grilled meats, and vegetarian meals.

18. Maintain Easy Access to Healthy Snacks: When hunger strikes, have wholesome snacks on hand to prevent grabbing less wholesome options.

Through the integration of these suggestions into your meal planning and preparation process, you may craft a well-rounded, savory, and anti-inflammatory diet that promotes your general health. Always remember to have fun and have an open mind while experimenting with different ingredients and recipes.

To discover your preferred flavors, try a variety of combinations.

- Juice and Zest of Citrus:

Zest and juice from citrus add brightness and taste. Orange, lemon, and lime can improve the flavor of marinades, salad dressings, and sauces.

- Deep Roasting:

Flavors can be enhanced by roasting proteins or veggies. Your food will taste richer and more fulfilling after the caramelization process.

- Make handmade dresses.

Utilizing herbs, balsamic vinegar, and olive oil, create your own dressings. You are able to maintain ingredient control and steer clear of the additional sugars present in certain store-bought dressings.

- Add vibrant vegetables.

To guarantee a varied nutrient profile, aim for a range of vibrant veggies. Carrots, bell peppers, tomatoes, and leafy greens may all add color to a meal.

- Dried and fresh herbs:

For layers of taste, use dried and fresh herbs. Dried herbs, such as oregano or thyme, can offer depth, while fresh herbs bring brightness.

- Season with Thought:

Moderately season your food so that the flavors of the ingredients themselves come through. If possible, use Himalayan or sea salt sparingly.

- Use spices in baking:

Use anti-inflammatory spices like nutmeg or cinnamon in baking recipes. This gives it some warmth and flavor without using too many added sweets.

- One-Pan or Sheet Pan Meals: Use one-pan or sheet pan meals to streamline your cooking. For a simple but tasty meal, roast a variety of veggies and protein combined with herbs and spices.
- Combine Anti-Inflammatory Smoothies: For a reviving and nutrient-dense smoothie, combine fruits such as berries, leafy greens, and flaxseeds or chia seeds.

- Hydrating Infusions: To make a tasty, hydrating beverage without additional sugars, infuse water with slices of cucumber, lemon, mint, or ginger.

- Careful Combining: Take into account complimentary tastes while combining components. For instance, combine salmon with a lemon-herb marinade or sweet potatoes with cinnamon.
- Employ Aromatics: Aromatics, such as shallots, garlic, and onions, can give your food more nuance and richness. When you first start cooking them, sauté them to build

taste.

- Harmony Sweet and Savory: Try striking a balance between flavors that are sweet and savory. For instance, a little honey or maple syrup can accentuate a dish's savory flavors.

Recall that the tastiest meals are frequently the ones that are easiest to prepare. To make delectable and anti-inflammatory recipes, concentrate on the inherent quality of your ingredients and the creative application of herbs and spices. Never be scared to use your imagination and modify recipes to your own tastes.

ANTI-INFLAMMATORY RECIPES FOR BREAKFAST

Simple and healthy anti-inflammatory breakfast ideas:

★ Blend frozen berries, bananas, Greek yogurt, and one teaspoon of turmeric to make a turmeric smoothie bowl. For extra taste, sprinkle almonds, seeds, and honey on top.

★Avocado Bread with Smoked Salmon: Top whole-grain bread with avocado mash. Add smoked salmon, chia seeds, and a squeeze of lemon juice on top for a breakfast that is high in nutrients.

★Chia Seed Pudding: Combine almond milk and chia seeds, then leave it overnight. Add some fresh berries, Greek yogurt, and anti-inflammatory cinnamon on top in the morning.

★Steel-cut oats cooked with almond milk go well with berries and nuts. Add some chopped nuts, mixed berries, and honey over top for a delicious and anti-inflammatory breakfast.

★Omelet of salmon and vegetables:

After whisking the eggs, add them to a pan. Add tomatoes, spinach, smoked salmon, and a small amount of turmeric. Toss into an omelet for a high-protein breakfast.

★Greek Yogurt Concession:

For a simple and delectable anti-inflammatory parfait, top Greek yogurt with fresh berries, low-sugar granola, and flaxseeds.

★ Breakfast Bowl with Quinoa:

After the quinoa is cooked, garnish it with almonds, banana slices, and honey. Quinoa makes a wholesome breakfast because it is high in protein and fiber.

★ Berry and Coconut Smoothie:

Smoothie: Blend together coconut milk, mixed berries, spinach, and protein powder; serve cold and soothe inflammation.

★ Whole Grain Toast with Berries and Almond Butter:

Toast with whole-grain bread spread with almond butter and topped with fresh berries. Antioxidants and good fats come together to provide a full breakfast.

★ Berry and Yogurt Parfait: Top plain yogurt with a medley of nuts, berries, and cinnamon. Probiotics and anti-inflammatory nutrients abound in this parfait.

★ Saute onions, bell peppers, and cubed sweet potatoes in olive oil to make a sweet potato breakfast hash. Add some fresh herbs and a fried or poached egg on top.

★ Berry and Spinach Smoothie: For a nutrient-dense and anti-inflammatory smoothie, blend spinach, mixed berries, bananas, and a scoop of protein powder with water or almond milk.

★ In a bowl, combine cottage cheese, sliced pineapple, kiwi, and a small amount of walnuts. Vitamins and minerals are added by the fruits, and cottage cheese supplies protein.

★ Muffins with Eggs and Veggies: Beat eggs and transfer to muffin liners. Add bell peppers, tomatoes, and spinach, all chopped. For a simple and convenient breakfast alternative, bake.

★ Mango Turmeric Overnight Oats: Mix together oats, chopped mango, almond milk, and a small amount of turmeric. After letting it set overnight, sprinkle the nuts and seeds on top in the morning.

In addition to being simple to make, these breakfast options are loaded with anti-inflammatory components to provide you with a nourishing start to the day. You are welcome to alter them to suit your dietary requirements and taste preferences.

ANTI-INFLAMMATORY RECIPES FOR LUNCH AND DINNER

Appetizing and Filling Anti-Inflammatory Meal and Supper Ideas:

**1. Quinoa and Salmon Bowl:

The dish consists of grilled salmon placed on top of cooked quinoa and a colorful mixture of roasted veggies, including bell peppers, broccoli, and cherry tomatoes. Add a drizzle of olive oil and top with chopped fresh herbs.

**2. Stir-fried Vegetable Chickpeas:

Sauté broccoli, snap peas, multicolored bell peppers, and chickpeas with garlic and olive oil. Add soy sauce, ginger, and turmeric for seasoning. Serve it with cauliflower or brown rice on the side.

**3. Grilled chicken over mixed greens:

Combine mixed greens, cucumber, cherry tomatoes, olives, and feta cheese in a salad. Add some grilled chicken on top, and drizzle some lemon and olive oil vinaigrette over it.

**4. Soup with Lentils and Vegetables:

Cook lentils in a vegetable broth with a variety of vegetables, such as kale, carrots, and celery. For extra taste, add coriander, cumin, and turmeric. Serve as a filling and inflammatory-reducing soup.

 **5. Curry with sweet potatoes and chickpeas:

Curry sauce made with coconut milk is cooked with chickpeas and sweet potatoes. Add coriander, cumin, and turmeric for seasoning. Serve with brown rice or quinoa.

**6. Vegetable and Cauliflower Pizza:

Make a cauliflower crust, then add tomato sauce, colorful veggies (such as bell peppers and spinach), and feta cheese or nutritional yeast on top.

**7. Vegetable and Tofu Skewers:

Tofu cubes and mixed vegetables should be marinated in a blend of herbs, garlic, and olive oil. Sew onto skewers and cook for a tasty, anti-inflammatory supper.

**8. Stuffed Chicken Breast with Spinach and Mushroom:

Stuff chicken breasts with a blend of garlic, mushrooms, and sautéed spinach. Once the chicken is thoroughly cooked, bake it and serve it with a

alongside roasted sweet potatoes or quinoa.

**9. Shrimp and Pesto Zucchini Noodles:

Noodles prepared from spiralized zucchini are served with a handmade pesto (olive oil, basil, pine nuts, and garlic). Add some sautéed shrimp on top for a tasty and light dinner.

**10. Turmeric and Ginger Chicken Stir-Fry: Add vibrant veggies like broccoli, bell peppers, and snap peas to stir-fried chicken. Add some ginger, turmeric, and low-sodium soy sauce for seasoning. Put it on top of cauliflower rice.

**11. Quinoa Salad with Black Beans, Avocado, and Chopped Tomatoes: Combine cooked quinoa, black beans, chopped tomato, and cilantro. Combine with a lime vinaigrette to create a cool, soothing salad.

**12. Turkey and Cabbage Skillet: Sauté onions, carrots, and shredded cabbage with ground turkey. For a simple and wholesome one-pan dinner, add some turmeric, cumin, and paprika for seasoning.

**13. Grilled Veggie Wrap: Grill bell peppers, zucchini, and eggplant, among other vegetables. Encase them in a whole-grain tortilla along with fresh herbs and hummus to create a filling and anti-inflammatory meal.

**14. Quinoa and Black Bean Stuffed Bell Peppers: Stuff cooked quinoa, black beans, corn, and tomatoes inside bell peppers. Serve the peppers with a dollop of Greek yogurt after baking them until they are soft.

**15. Curry with Eggplant and Chickpeas: Marinate eggplant and chickpeas in a curry sauce flavored with tomatoes, coconut milk, cumin, and turmeric. Put it on top of basmati rice.

In addition to being tasty, these dishes include anti-inflammatory substances to improve your general health. You are welcome to alter them to suit your dietary requirements and tastes.

Anti-inflammatory lunch and dinner that are well-balanced and delicious:

★Quinoa, roasted vegetables, and grilled salmon:

Components:

Filets of salmonQuinoaVegetable mixture (bell peppers, broccoli, and cherry tomatoes)Olive oilfresh herbs, like dill or parsley   slices of lemonPowdered garlicGingerTo taste, add salt and pepper.

Guidelines:

To prepare the quinoa, follow the directions on the package. Using a fork, fluff and set aside.

Marinate salmon by rubbing salmon fillets with a mixture of olive oil, salt, pepper, turmeric, and garlic powder. Give it a minimum of fifteen minutes to marinate.

Grill Prep: Turn up the heat to medium-high on the grill or grill pan.

Grill Salmon: Grill salmon until it achieves your preferred doneness, around 4–5 minutes per side. Generously squeeze lemon juice onto the fillets.

Roast Vegetables: Combine olive oil, salt, and pepper and toss with mixed vegetables. Bake or broil them until they are soft and beginning to take on some color.

Assemble Plate: Arrange quinoa on a platter and top with roasted veggies and grilled fish. For extra taste, sprinkle some fresh herbs over top.

★ Brown rice, vegetables, and chickpeas stir-fried:

Components:

Cooked or canned chickpeasmixed veggies, including broccoli, snap peas, and bell pepperscooked brown riceOlive oilGarlicGingerSalt-free soy sauceGingerOil from sesame (optional)As a garnish, use green onions.

Guidelines:

Prepare the ingredients: if using canned chickpeas, rinse and drain them. Chop the ginger, garlic, and mixed vegetables.

To sauté aromatics, heat up some olive oil in a big wok or skillet. Add the minced ginger and garlic, and cook for one minute, or until fragrant.

Stir-fry veggies: Put a mixture of veggies in the skillet and cook, stirring occasionally, until the vegetables are crisp but just slightly soft.

Add chickpeas: Cook the chickpeas for a further two to three minutes after adding them to the vegetables.

Add Soy Sauce and Turmeric: Drizzle the mixture with low-sodium soy sauce and sprinkle with turmeric. Stir well to ensure an even coating. For added taste, feel free to add a few drops of sesame oil.

Serve over brown rice: Arrange cooked brown rice on a bed of chickpeas and veggie stir-fry. Add chopped green onions as a garnish.

To serve, divide the quinoa salad with a Mediterranean flair onto plates and start serving right away.

With an abundance of vibrant veggies, nutritious grains, and lean proteins in balance, these dishes also have anti-inflammatory flavors and ingredients. To suit your nutritional requirements and tastes, adjust the serving proportions.

SNACKS AND SIDES

Snack Ideas That Are Good for an Anti-Inflammatory Diet:

- Smoothie with Mixed Berries: Blend together Greek yogurt, strawberries, raspberries, and blueberries with a small amount of almond milk. For an additional anti-inflammatory benefit, add a dash of turmeric.
- Avocado and Tomato Salsa: Finely chop ripe avocados and combine them with lime juice, cherry tomatoes, red onion, and cilantro. Accompany with cucumber slices or whole-grain crackers.
- Roasted Nuts with Turmeric: Combine almonds with a small amount of olive oil, turmeric, and a dash of black pepper. Bake until golden, then savor as a crispy, pain-relieving snack.
- Greek Yogurt Parfait: For a high-protein and nutrient-dense parfait, top Greek yogurt with fresh berries, honey, and flaxseeds or chia seeds.

- ★ Hummus and Veggie Sticks: Dip bell pepper, cucumber, and carrot sticks into store-bought or homemade hummus. A good source of olive oil and chickpeas is found in hummus.
- ★ Chia Seed Pudding: Combine almond milk and chia seeds, allowing them to soak all night. Add sliced mango and kiwi to the top for a delicious, anti-inflammatory pudding.
- ★ Roasted Chickpeas: Dredge chickpeas in olive oil and season with paprika, cumin, and a tiny bit of turmeric.
- ★ Crispy roasting makes for a filling, high-protein snack. To make kale chips, gently massage the leaves of the kale leaves with a little olive oil and nutritional yeast. A crunchy and wholesome substitute for potato chips is to bake them until they become crispy.
- ★ Make a fresh fruit salad by combining different fresh fruits, such as berries, pineapple, and oranges. Squeeze in some lime juice and add some mint for a cool, anti-inflammatory snack.
- ★ Pineapple Cottage Cheese: Savor a dish of cottage cheese with chunks of juicy pineapple on top.

Protein is provided by cottage cheese, while natural sweetness is added by pineapple.

★ Almond butter on sliced apples: Cut apples into thin slices and coat them with almond butter. A balance of fiber, good fats, and anti-inflammatory substances is provided by this combo.

★ Edamame Pods: Steam the edamame pods and then lightly season with sea salt. Edamame is a fantastic plant-based source of fiber and protein.

★ Almonds and Dark Chocolate: Assemble a small portion of almonds and dark chocolate (70% cocoa or more). Almonds offer good lipids, and dark chocolate has antioxidants.

★ Turmeric Tea: Prepare a cup of turmeric tea by adding some ginger and honey to it. This hot tea makes a calming, anti-inflammatory snack.

★ Cucumber Slices with Guacamole: Dredge cucumber slices in guacamole that has tomatoes, onions, cilantro, and ripe avocados.

A filling and healthy snack.

In addition to being tasty, these snacks contain substances that have been shown to have anti-inflammatory qualities. Include these in your diet for savory and nourishing snacks in between meals.

Delicious Side Dishes to Go with Main Courses That Are Nutritious and Wholesome:

1. Quinoa and Veggie Pilaf: Cook the quinoa and combine it with cherry tomatoes, zucchini, and bell peppers that have been sautéed. Add some lemon juice, olive oil, and fresh herbs for seasoning.
2. Roasted Sweet Potato Wedges: Finely chop sweet potatoes and combine them with paprika, olive oil, and a small amount of cinnamon. For an intensely tasty and nutrient-rich side, roast until caramelized.
3. Garlic Sauteed Spinach: Finely chop your garlic and sauté it with some fresh spinach in olive oil until it wilts. Add a squeeze of lemon juice, salt, and pepper for a fast and nutrient-dense side dish.
4. Mash Cauliflower: Steam the cauliflower and mash it with a little garlic, olive oil, and fresh herbs. A low-carb substitute for mashed potatoes that is high in vitamins and fiber.
5. Quinoa Salad with Almonds and Cranberries: Toss cooked quinoa with almond slivers, minced parsley,

and dried cranberries. Toss with a mild vinaigrette for a nutritious and revitalizing side dish.

6. Roast Brussels sprouts in olive oil until they get crispy, and serve with a balsamic glaze. For a tasty and wholesome side, add a balsamic glaze and some toasted walnuts on top.

7. Brown rice infused with turmeric: To add color and reduce inflammation, cook brown rice with a small pinch of turmeric. For freshness, add chopped cilantro and lime zest.

8. To make a caprese salad, arrange fresh mozzarella, sliced tomatoes, and basil leaves on a dish. For a traditional and filling side, drizzle with extra virgin olive oil and balsamic glaze.

9. Lemon-Roasted Asparagus: Dredge asparagus spears in olive oil, then roast them until they are soft. For a zesty and tasty side, squeeze some fresh lemon juice over the top and top with grated Parmesan.

10. Roast or steam butternut squash, then mash it with a small amount of butter or olive oil. Add nutmeg, salt, and pepper for seasoning, and you have a nourishing and satisfying dish.

11.   Cucumber and Chickpea Salad: Mix feta cheese, cherry tomatoes, chopped cucumbers, and red onion with the chickpeas. Toss with lemon juice, olive oil, and a dash of oregano.

12.   Toss cooked lentils with cherry tomatoes, cucumber, red onion, and feta cheese to make a lentil and tomato salad. Serve with a mild vinaigrette for a delicious and protein-rich side.

13.   How to Make Baked Acorn Squash Rings:

Acorn squash should be cut into rings, brushed with olive oil, and sprinkled with cinnamon before baking. For a flavorful and sweet side dish, bake until soft.

14. Nuts, chopped nuts, and fresh herbs are combined with cooked wild rice and dried cranberries. A pleasant and filling side featuring a variety of textures.

15. Eggplant and Tomato Bake: Arrange tomatoes and eggplant slices thickly in a baking dish. After adding some Italian herbs and a drizzle of olive oil, bake until soft and golden.

These side dishes not only go well with main courses, but they also add vital nutrients and a range of flavors and textures. You are welcome to combine them in any way to make a balanced and filling dinner that suits your tastes.

DESSERTS AND TREATS

Recipes for decadent but healthful desserts:

- Make dark chocolate avocado mousse by blending ripe avocados with vanilla extract, unsweetened cocoa powder, and a small amount of maple syrup. For a luscious, creamy chocolate dessert, chill the mousse.
- Baked Apples with Walnuts and Cinnamon: Core the apples, then stuff the center with granulated cinnamon, walnuts, and honey. Bake for a warm, satisfying dessert, or until the apples are soft.

- Chia Seed Pudding Parfait: Arrange a layer of fresh berries, Greek yogurt, and chia seed pudding. Add some granola on top for some crunch and sweetness.
- Freeze banana slices after dipping them in melted dark chocolate until the chocolate solidifies. This makes frozen banana bites. A natural sweetness in a straightforward and delicious treat.
- Coconut and Berry Nice Cream: Process coconut milk and frozen mixed berries till smooth. Serve as a naturally sweetened, dairy-free substitute for ice cream.
- Greek Yogurt and Honey Berries Bowl: Mix Greek yogurt with a variety of berries and pour honey over the mixture. A handful of chopped nuts can be added for a decadent and high-protein dessert.
- Dates with Almond Butter Stuffed: Take out the dates' pits and stuff them with a tiny dollop of almond butter. A delicious blend of creaminess and sweetness.
- Rolling oats, pumpkin puree, nut butter, honey, and a mixture of pumpkin spices are combined to make pumpkin spice energy balls. For a tasty and

invigorating dessert, roll into energy balls and place in the refrigerator.

- Almonds dusted with cocoa powder: Combine almonds with a small amount of sea salt and unsweetened cocoa powder.

Roast until crispy in the oven for a filling and chocolatey snack.

- For the sweet potato chocolate brownies, mash the sweet potatoes and mix with some cocoa powder, almond flour, and maple syrup. For a fudgy and guilt-free dessert, bake brownies.
- Avocado Chocolate Truffles: Process ripe avocados until smooth, then roll the consistency into truffle-sized spheres using dark chocolate. For a sophisticated and healthier truffle option, coat with cocoa powder.
- Blend a variety of frozen berries with a squeeze of lime juice to make a mixed-berry sorbet. For a naturally sweet and pleasant sorbet, freeze the ingredients.
- Protein-Packed Chocolate Smoothie Bowl: Process almond milk, chocolate protein powder, and frozen

banana in a blender. For a bowl full of nutrients, garnish with almond butter, chopped strawberries, and nuts.

- Chia seeds, almond milk, and a sprinkling of vanilla flavor are combined to make vanilla chia seed pudding with mango. For a delightful and tropical dessert, sprinkle diced mango on top.
- For the cinnamon-baked pears, slice the pears and mix in a small amount of honey and cinnamon. For a naturally sweet dish that is warm and cozy, bake until soft.

These dessert ideas provide a satisfying finish to your meals without sacrificing nutrition in favor of enjoyment and wellness. Eat these sweets guilt-free as part of a balanced, healthy diet.

Providing Your Sweet Thirst Without Giving Up on Anti-Inflammatory Principles:

Take pleasure in a warm latte infused with ginger, turmeric, and a dash of almond milk—the Turmeric Golden Milk Latte. For a soothing, anti-inflammatory drink, mildly sweeten with honey or maple syrup.

Baked Apple Slices with Cinnamon: Cut apples into slices and sprinkle with cinnamon. For a naturally sweet and comforting dish without extra sweeteners, bake until soft.

Greek yogurt should be layered with fresh mixed berries and chia seeds for a mixed-berry yogurt parfait. Pour over some honey for a filling and anti-inflammatory treat.

Melted dark chocolate should be poured over fresh strawberries to create a delicious treat. When consumed in moderation as part of an anti-inflammatory diet, dark chocolate can be enjoyed because it contains antioxidants.

Chia Seed Pudding with Berries: In a bowl, combine chia seeds and almond milk; stir and allow to thicken. Add a variety of berries on top for a tasty and nutrient-rich treat.

Frozen Grapes: As a naturally sweet and refreshing snack, freeze grapes. They are a tasty alternative to popsicles loaded with sugar.

Pineapple and Mint Sorbet: For a naturally sweet and refreshing sorbet, blend frozen pineapple with a few mint leaves. There is no need for additional sweets.

Coconut Date Rolls: Process dates in a food processor with unsweetened shredded coconut. Form them into little balls for a naturally sweet treat that is chewy and pleasant.

Mango Turmeric Smoothie: Process the mango, coconut water, ginger, and turmeric in a blender. It's a tasty and nutritious dessert choice because of the anti-inflammatory components and tropical flavors.

Almond Butter Banana Bites: Spread banana slices with almond butter, then place them one on top of the other. Cravings for sweetness are satiated by the mix of sweet banana and creamy almond butter.

TIPS FOR SUCCESS

Useful Advice for Maintaining an Anti-Inflammatory Lifestyle Consistency:

1. Become knowledgeable: Find out more about the advantages of eating foods that reduce inflammation. Knowing the guiding principles of your lifestyle might inspire you to make wise decisions.

2. Gradual Changes: Make adjustments bit by bit. It might be stressful to try to change your diet drastically all at once. Make minor changes at first, then expand on them.

3. Meal Planning: Arrange your food in advance to guarantee that it has a range of nutrient-dense, anti-inflammatory components. This lessens the possibility of choosing quick but unhealthy solutions.

The perimeter of the grocery store is typically where you'll find lean proteins, nutritious grains, and fresh produce, so use this strategy when grocery shopping. Reduce the number of inflammatory and processed foods on your shopping list.

4. Cook at Home: Make as many meals as you can in your own kitchen. You can now choose the ingredients and cooking techniques you choose, resulting in a more anti-inflammatory meal.

5. Investigate new dishes: Keeping your meals interesting can be achieved by investigating new dishes that adhere to anti-inflammatory principles. This gives your eating options more variation and keeps you from getting bored.

6. Consciously Consuming Food: By observing your body's signals of hunger and fullness, cultivate mindful eating. In addition to promoting a healthier connection with food, this helps avoid overeating.

7. Hydration is important. Drink plenty of water, herbal teas, and fruit- and herb-infused water to stay hydrated. Maintaining adequate hydration promotes general health and may help lead to a lifestyle free from inflammation.

8. Include anti-inflammatory spices and herbs. To improve the flavor of your food, try experimenting with herbs and spices like turmeric, ginger, garlic, and cinnamon that have anti-inflammatory qualities.

9. Equilibrated Dish: Aim for a colorful, well-balanced plate that has a good amount of veggies, lean meats, and healthy grains. This guarantees a wide variety of nutrients. Examine the labels: Read food labels carefully to find out about added sugars, harmful fats, and other ingredients. Make a minimal choice.

10. Social Assistance:

Tell your loved ones about your experience using anti-inflammatory foods. Having a network of support can boost confidence and improve quality of life.

11. Frequent Workout:

Make physical activity a regular part of your schedule. Exercise promotes general wellbeing and has been linked to anti-inflammatory effects.

12. Body-Mind Techniques:

Incorporate techniques for lowering stress, such as yoga, meditation, or deep breathing. These techniques can help control stress levels, which can help reduce inflammation caused by chronic stress.

13. Track Development:

Maintain a journal to document any changes in your general well-being, mood, and energy levels as you make improvements. Reward minor accomplishments to maintain motivation.

14. Expert Advice:

Speak with a trained dietician or healthcare provider to create an anti-inflammatory plan that works for your specific requirements and health objectives.

15. Culinary Exploration: Try a range of cuisines and discover meals from around the world that inherently adhere to anti-inflammatory concepts. This makes your meals more exciting.

Treat yourself with kindness. Recognize that excellence is not the aim. If you do occasionally stray from your goal, treat yourself with kindness and put your attention back on choosing better options going forward.

Adopting an anti-inflammatory lifestyle is a journey, and consistency is crucial. These useful suggestions might help you establish long-lasting routines that promote your general health and wellbeing.

CONCLUSION

For those who are unfamiliar with anti-inflammatory cooking, the "Beginner's Guide to Anti-Inflammatory

Cookbooks" offers a thorough synopsis of key ideas. Among the essential ideas are:

Overview of Anti-Inflammatory Eating: recognizing the basic ideas behind an anti-inflammatory diet and stressing the role that food plays in lowering inflammation and improving general health.

Basic Anti-Inflammatory Foods: Choosing and utilizing essential anti-inflammatory foods, like fruits, vegetables, lean meats, and healthy fats, to lay the groundwork for wholesome meals.

Herbs and Spices for Inflammation: This article explores the potent anti-inflammatory qualities of herbs and spices, emphasizing the use of components like garlic, ginger, turmeric, and others in regular recipes.

Meal Planning and Preparation Strategies: Useful advice for efficient grocery shopping, meal planning, and cooking methods to create a fun and sustainable anti-inflammatory diet.

The balanced nutrition approach places a strong emphasis on the value of a plate that is well-balanced and contains a range of nutrients from various food groups in order to promote general health and wellbeing.

Practices for Mindful Eating: fostering awareness of hunger and fullness, encouraging attention during meals, and developing a healthy relationship with food.

Hydration and Lifestyle Factors: Recognizing the importance of maintaining an anti-inflammatory lifestyle through appropriate hydration, frequent exercise, stress reduction, and enough sleep.

Examining Anti-Inflammatory Cookbooks: Offering advice on choosing and using anti-inflammatory cookbooks, as well as a variety of recipes and recipe ideas for individuals who are unfamiliar with this type of cooking.

Tracking Development and Celebrating Success: Motivating people to follow their path toward an anti-inflammatory lifestyle by keeping track of their development, acknowledging minor victories, and maintaining motivation.

Seeking Professional Guidance: Understanding the importance of speaking with registered dietitians or other healthcare professionals to receive individualized guidance based on each person's unique health needs and objectives.

Diverse gastronomic exploration: increasing the pleasure of meals by promoting gastronomic diversity through the exploration of other cuisines and international foods that are in line with anti-inflammatory principles.

Flexibility and self-compassion: stressing the value of these qualities and realizing that leading an anti-inflammatory lifestyle is a gradual process that allows for personal preferences and modifications.

This comprehensive beginner's guide offers a range of useful information, including dietary recommendations, lifestyle advice, and practical insights to help people embrace and sustain an anti-inflammatory diet.

Dear Readers,

You're about to go on a voyage of anti-inflammatory cooking that will change your life! Equipped with the potency of nutrient-dense foods, you're ready to set out on a journey that will nourish your body from the inside out while simultaneously tantalizing your taste senses.

Do not be alarmed by the intricacy; this is an exploration voyage, not a competition. Start with basic,healthy items such as whole grains, colorful fruits, and veggies. These gems possess the anti-inflammatory properties your body longs for, in addition to their delicious flavor.

Your sous chef is confidence, and your secret ingredient is enthusiasm. Accept the colorful range of spices, such as ginger and turmeric, which not only provide flavor to your food but also have strong anti-inflammatory effects.

Every recipe in your kitchen is an experiment in self-care; your kitchen is a laboratory of wellbeing. Give in to the excitement of exploration and enjoy each mouthful as a step toward a more vibrant, healthier version of yourself.

Put on your apron, sharpen your cutlery, and enjoy your kitchen as the delicious sound of anti-inflammatory food sizzles. This is a journey about embracing a lifestyle that nourishes and revitalizes, not simply about cooking. Cheers to a future of well-seasoned health and happy cooking!

Good appetite!

www.ingramcontent.com/pod-product-compliance
Lightning Source LLC
Chambersburg PA
CBHW060950260726

48661CB00005B/1827